WiseTeenz

Faith-Based Health
Education for Teen Girls

Wise Teenz

Faith-Based Health Education for Teen Girls

SULEIKA JUST-BUDDY MICHEL, MD, F.A.C.O.G.

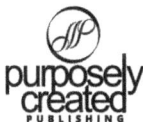

purposely created
PUBLISHING

Special discounts are available on bulk quantity purchases by book clubs, associations and special interest groups. For details email: sales@publishyourgift.com or call (888) 949-6228.

For information log on to www.PublishYourGift.com

This book is dedicated to Ricardo, Laila, and Jadon, my living heartbeats. I thank my husband, Ricardo, for his love and patience over the last twenty-two years. I thank my favorite daughter, Laila, for being the impetus to create this gift to share with the world. I thank my favorite son, Jadon, whose laugh and smile brighten my day on a regular basis. I also dedicate my first book especially to my mom, the one who inspired me to always push beyond expectations. Thank you to my family, friends, Sorors, patients, and colleagues who encouraged this ambitious venture. Pastor Mike Robinson, your input and prayer on this book is appreciated more than you could ever know. Thank you to Dr. Drai for your direction in transforming my life and pushing me to pursue my purpose. Thank you, God, for the vision, discipline, and open doors that allowed this passion to be poured onto paper. Grateful.

Table of Contents

Introduction

Since I was in medical school, I have found that I enjoy speaking to and educating girls about their bodies. While facilitating health classes for girls at local Christian schools, I asked them where they obtained their information about their bodies. Unanimously they all answered, "The internet." When I asked them what they were typing into the search engine to get answers, they stated, "Vagina... breasts..." They added that they had to be extra careful because those prompts inadvertently expose them to inappropriate images. They were attempting to get answers to benign questions but were clearly accidently falling into an internet black hole of situations and images designated for adult eyes only.

The purpose of this book is to provide high school girls with information about their bodies in a safe space. This faith-based message is designed to make you more confident and knowledgeable about your temple. An educated girl in Christ becomes a transformed light for the world.

---

1 Corinthians 8:3, NIV

"But whoever loves God is known by God."

Foreword

By Rev. Michael Robinson, MS Counseling

Romans 8:5-6, NIV

"Those who live according to the flesh have their minds set on what the flesh desires; but those who live in accordance with the Spirit have their minds set on what the Spirit desires. The mind governed by the flesh is death, *but the mind governed by the Spirit is life and peace.*"

Most fathers would walk through fire, climb the tallest mountain, and swim shark infested waters just to put a smile on their daughter's face. I'm like that with my precious little teenage princess, Joy. But when it comes to dads dealing with their daughter's puberty and other feminine issues of life, many dads cower, cringe, and crumble like Superman exposed to kryptonite!

I am not a fan of the Kardashian women, but I do love a quote that sister Khloe shared about girls going through puberty: "I just think that knowing about your body at any age, whether it's educating yourself on fertility, getting mammograms, going through puberty - whatever it may be, is really important. I just really encourage women empowerment and being comfortable talking about these issues."

Puberty for teenage girls can be some of the most harrowing, challenging, and awkward years. As a concerned dad, I want to be an informed and available parent to help my daughter navigate the murky waters of puberty by empowering her with the right information at the right time. And as a concerned urban pastor, I want to be able to provide tweens and teenage girls in my church congregation (and the community at-large) with credible resource information that can empower them to make positive life choices about their health, sexuality, fertility, and spiritual well-being.

WiseTeenz is an audacious resource book that addresses many sensitive and confidential feminine issues that tweens and teenage girls wrestle with on a daily basis. *WiseTeenz* was written by my friend and medical doctor, Dr. Suleika Just-Buddy Michel. She wrote this book as a vital source to educate tween and teen girls with medical, fact-based information presented in understandable language that is easily relatable. This book is the perfect tool for concerned parents, teachers, medical doctors, mentors, and ministry leaders. It really is an excellent option for all who need a credible health resource that is intentionally aimed at tweens and teen girls.

I've known Dr. Michel for over twenty years, during her undergrad years, her years through medical school, as well as the completion of her OBGYN residency program. We first met during my years working as a Recruiting/ Training Staff Specialist with INROADS/ Philadelphia, Inc., a national award-winning leadership development organization for highly talented minority collegians. She was a stellar scholar with an evident bright future, and the girl can dance, too! I take partial credit for connecting this member of Delta Sigma Theta Sorority, Inc., with her husband Ricardo Michel (a brilliant finance guru). They were the hip, young, power couple as undergrads with INROADS. I love them both dearly. Their philanthropy, strong parental bond with their children, and commitment to help others level up is truly awe-inspiring.

Dr. Michel graduated from the world-renowned Johns Hopkins University in Baltimore, Maryland. She currently works in Annapolis, Maryland, where she is a partner in a group OBGYN practice. Dr. Michel is using her medical expertise in *family planning*, *obstetrics*, and *gynecology* to equip girls with the information needed to make informed decisions about their unique feminine health.

I esteem Dr. Michel for her foresight to produce relevant and informative social media video blogs that solely focus on feminine issues that concern young girls. In writing this book, Dr. Michel has provided yet another safe, informative, and engaging platform filling tweens and teenage girls with vital information that will help them successfully navigate through the murky waters of puberty. In addition, it addresses sensitive topics concerning the female anatomy, sexuality, emotions, and other pertinent female concerns. Without the proper guidance, information, and positive support, the stress of such radical life and body changes can become overwhelming for some girls.

Thankfully, Dr. Michel's *WiseTeenz* makes this daunting personal journey for tween and teen girls more governable. In the Bible, the wisdom book of Proverbs 4:7 says, *"Wisdom is the principal thing; therefore get wisdom: and with all thy getting get understanding."* May *WiseTeenz* become a go-to resource, blessing all girls seeking wisdom and understanding about their unique and complicated femininity. To God be the glory and blessings to all.

About Rev. Michael Smi Robinson, MS Counseling

Rev. Robinson is an award-winning college administrator at Temple University, a local columnist for Scoop USA newspaper, and a celebrated business leader –winner of the prestigious *Industry Icon Award* in Philadelphia, PA. He serves as the ordained Senior Pastor of Greater Enon Missionary Baptist Church, 1854 N. 22nd Street, Philadelphia, PA 19121. He's happily married to his wife, Dana, and they have two active teens, Joy and Matthew.

PARTS OF YOUR TEMPLE

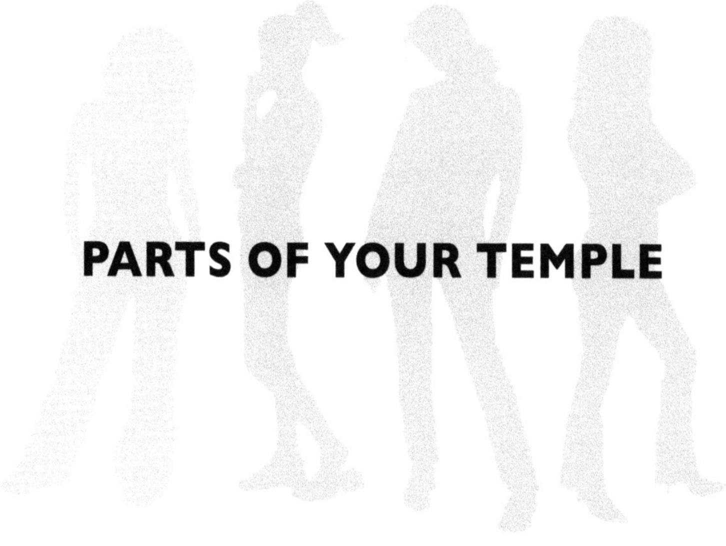

I. The Head

MINDSET

It has been said that the body of a fish rots from the head down. In other words, the decomposition process of the entire body of the fish starts at the top. This, too, applies in many ways to the human body regarding your mindset. The head controls bodily functions *directly* through numerous neurological pathways. It controls the body *indirectly* through thoughts. There are miraculous anecdotes illustrating how thoughts change the course of medical catastrophes, outcomes of athletic games, business and personal goals, among other life occurrences. Positive thoughts promote growth. Negative thoughts can promote decay. Your thoughts also have the ability to govern how the rest of your body responds to situations, but even more powerful, they can *change situations around you*, so you can function optimally. Throw out that rotten, negative mindset, so you can thrive and change the world, while allowing it to also change you in a positive way.

According to *USA Today*, a study of pediatric hospitals, released in May 2017, found that the number of patients, ages five to seventeen, admitted for suicidal thoughts and actions, more than doubled from the years 2008 to 2015. The Centers for Disease Control and Prevention have found that the suicide rate for white children and teens between the ages of ten and seventeen was up seventy percent between 2006 and 2016. The group at highest risk for suicide was white males between the ages of fourteen and twenty-one. Although black children and teens kill themselves less often than white youth do, the rate of increase was higher, a tragic seventy-seven percent.

We can be our own worst enemy, filling our heads with cyclic mantras of doubt, in an unconscious effort to reaffirm that we are not good enough. I challenge you to break that cycle by exchanging thoughts promoting decay and stagnancy to thoughts and images that inspire a growth mindset with increased forward momentum. Where do you start? With prayer, of course. God is very informal and always available. You don't need to meet Him only in church. He will come to you whenever and wherever you need Him. Just ask. Allow Him to fill your head with positive, productive, confidence-building verbiage that reminds you that you are indeed good enough because after all, He made you. Change your mental script to something that encourages you to be the best you can be. It's not easy, but it's definitely possible over time. Learn to make self-motivation a habit. It's a valuable tool that can be used well into adulthood.

Ecclesiastes 11:4-6, NLT

"Farmers who wait for perfect weather never plant. If they watch every cloud, they never harvest. Just as you cannot understand the path of the wind or the mystery of a tiny baby growing in its mother's womb, so you cannot understand the activity of God, who does all things. Plant your seeds in the morning and keep busy all afternoon, for you don't know if profit will come from one activity or another– or maybe both."

Are you afraid of planting something because everything isn't "perfect?" Do you find yourself getting distracted by a fear of failure? Maybe you're delaying a tryout for a sport's team or a part in a play because you think you should master their requirements first so you'll be chosen. Are you afraid to create a personal best goal in a sport because you think you might never accomplish it? Perhaps you are afraid to try to lose weight because you don't feel you have enough time to exercise and don't have enough willpower to manage a healthy diet consistently. Do you want to create an object, paint a beautiful picture, or travel abroad, but you're concerned about limited ability and financial resources? You must start somewhere. And I'll let you in on a little secret – you don't have to be perfect when you start.

Plant already. Try out for that sport. Write down your goals for personal best successes to stay accountable. For example, if you're interested in a semester abroad, start researching those travel programs. When you make up your mind to do something that God has placed on your heart, doors open. Opportunities abound. What you think about and focus on gets bigger, but don't just *think* about your desires and goals. Do the work to make them happen. Get ready and stay ready for the time when opportunity meets preparation and decides to pursue a long-term relationship. The universe has a way of conforming to the plan of bringing life to your gifts, especially when He is in charge. Your mindset can make or break you. Don't be that rotting fish.

Change your mindset.

You are young. You have many years ahead of you. Author a new cognitive dialogue if yours is one of fear, doubt, self-sabotage, or self-harm. Plant your ideas and goals, water them, and watch them flourish. Be grateful for small miracles linking together for a larger vision. Try something new. Step out of fear. Be your own biggest cheerleader. Stop the negative talk to yourself about your friendships, body image, grades, athletic ability, artistic prowess, musical talent, or whatever the issue may be. If you feel like you're unable to get out of a negative rut, don't be afraid to seek help from a trusted adult or even a professional counselor. Rise, conquer, and be great.

VISION

Habakkuk 2:2, NIV

"Then the Lord replied: 'Write down the revelation and make it plain on tablets so that a herald may run with it.'"

The eyes are a roadmap to one's soul. Whatever your eyes feast upon can get absorbed into your very being. By this age, you know right from wrong. You are fully aware of which images are for your eyes and those that go against God's desire for you. Be careful what you allow your eyes to land upon. Imagery and experiences have a way of finding a home in your mind and spirit.

How is your vision, literally? Are you able to see the board in school, or is the writing blurry? Do you get headaches after reading for long periods of time? Address visual impairments early. Mention any concerns to a parent or guardian and be sure to make an appointment with an ophthalmologist or optometrist to make your vision as clear as possible. You should have your vision checked every year if you are under the age of eighteen, and every two years from age eighteen through forty. Don't be embarrassed about glasses or contacts. Be the trendsetter by getting an eclectic pair of frames for those eyes of yours. Make a fashion statement. Do whatever you need to do to have ideal vision.

And then, how is your *vision*? Are you setting goals? It's always a good habit to write down short-term and long-term goals. Set goals for the quarter, semester, and your entire academic year. Think about where you would like to be and what you would like to be doing in three years, five years, or ten years. Make a vision board. In fact, consider having a vision board party with friends to get everyone focused on their own talents, passions, and journeys to fulfilling their dreams.

Are you looking at situations and experiences solely with your own eyes, or are you examining those things through God's lens? Envision yourself and the satisfaction you will feel after accomplishing your specific goals. Break large tasks down to bite-sized pieces to make completion more realistic. For example, if you play a sport and have a personal goal for the season or year, figure out what you need to do in each of your practices to make that happen. Put in the work. Keep reminding yourself that God has given you a gift. He will open doors for your gift to grow when you not only believe in Him but also believe in yourself.

"Don't compare your life to others. There's no comparison between the sun and the moon. They both shine when it's their time."

—Unknown

Short Term Goals

_____

_____

_____

_____

_____

_____

_____

_____

_____

_____

_____

_____

_____

_____

_____

_____

_____

_____

_____

_____

Short Term Goals

_____

_____

_____

_____

_____

_____

_____

_____

_____

_____

_____

_____

_____

_____

_____

_____

_____

_____

Long Term Goals

Long Term Goals

_____

_____

_____

_____

_____

_____

_____

_____

_____

_____

_____

_____

_____

_____

_____

_____

_____

_____

EARS

---

2 Samuel 22:7, NIV

"In my distress I called to the Lord; I called out to my God. From his temple He heard my voice; my cry came to his ears."

God hears your prayers. When you feel you have no one else to turn to, His ears are always open. You just need to make time to listen for His answer. Too much noise can keep you from hearing a blessing.

Your ears are essentially another pathway for everything outside in the world to enter your brain. The sense of hearing can be more powerful than sight for many. It has such power that it allows the blind to be in tune with the subtleties of their surroundings. They are able to navigate the environment by using their auditory (hearing) system to locate sources and sound-reflecting objects (echo reflection). Whenever you can, safeguard your ears. You'll appreciate that effort when you get older.

Who else do you listen to? As a teen maturing into a young adult, sometimes it seems like you know more than those seasoned adults in your life. In some cases, that may be true. Hopefully, advice from your friends and society doesn't always outweigh advice from those adults close to you, who are legitimately trying to shower you with knowledge based on personal experience. Keep in mind, though, now is also a time when parents may not be your only source for necessary life information. You must figure out who to trust and how to get answers to questions safely.

Many times, parents provide rules and recommendations in an attempt to keep you from making the same mistakes they may have made as a young adult. Why would you want to jump unknowingly into a pool of scalding hot water when you have someone who can say, "Hey, I jumped into that same body of water, and I got severely burned? I'd stay away from that if I were you." If you don't have involved parents, consider another trusted adult as an advisor or simply a sounding board. Also, appreciate that most times any advice given by an adult is given from a protective heart. Listen with an open heart. Just as He wants to keep you from harm, your earthly parents also take that role very seriously.

In some situations, you may hear more of what your friends have to say than what a trusted adult says. Be sure you have friends in your circle who not only have your best interests at heart, but who also, most of all, have similar values. Values and religion are two very different principles and, in some cases, are mutually exclusive. Just because a friend attends the same church as you or is a member of a similar church denomination, it doesn't mean you share the same values and vice-versa. Choose your circle based on your value system. You are not an experiment. Do not listen to so-called friends who encourage you to try out something that is known or unknown to cause harm or addiction. Be leery of advice from strangers. Seek medical advice from a professional rather than "Dr. Google." If it sounds crazy, it probably is crazy. This really is common sense, but you'd be surprised how many people find themselves in precarious predicaments by not following the basic tenets of sound judgment.

Be intentional with what you place in your ears for motivation, pleasure, or focus. Music, in particular, has been proven to affect brain waves. If you are a music lover, compile a variety of playlists to go along with your assignments and activities. My own playlists for my workouts at the gym are nothing at all like the playlists I use while working or writing. Be cautious with the volume, so it doesn't exacerbate the natural hearing loss that comes with age. Listening to extremely loud music, particularly with devices directly on or in your ears, can cause hearing loss to occur earlier in life. Use music as a catalyst for something good. It may spark energy, hone focus, or induce sleep. Your body needs all three so achieving them is considered success.

MOUTH

Proverbs 16:24, NIV

"Gracious words are a honeycomb, sweet to the soul and healing to the bones."

Treating others with respect, using your words and tone, should become second nature, something you don't think twice about because it flows from you naturally. What have you been talking about lately? Is gossip part of your active speech? How do you speak to your friends, your parents, other elders, or yourself? How you address adults can be a predictor of how you'll respond in other interactions. Be purposeful, but gentle, when expressing your opinions. Your delivery can close ears or open hearts.

Gossip is a waste of time. Spend your energy on topics that are true and uplifting. Speak life into situations, literally, through prayer and verbal affirmations. When you're around

> *"Great minds discuss ideas.*
> *Average minds discuss events.*
> *Small minds discuss people."*
>
> **—Eleanor Roosevelt**

others, remember people don't need to know everything that you're thinking. If it's not kind, keep it to yourself unless it's solicited. Kindness bridges different perspectives on issues. It can create a space open to disclosing and discussing differences of opinion without being verbally harmful. You don't have to agree with everyone's opinions but listening to opposing ideas on topics can shed more light on and even confirm some of your own beliefs. Words have energy. Use that energy in a positive way.

Maya Angelou wrote in her book, *Letter to My Daughter*, "We need to have the courage to say that obesity is not funny and vulgarity is not amusing. Insolent children and submissive parents are not the characters we want to admire and emulate. Flippancy and sarcasm are not the qualities we need to include in our daily conversation."

Words should be used to uplift. Be careful what words you allow to be released from your mouth. You cannot take back what you verbally place into the atmosphere, whether it is spoken directly to another person, in text, or even posted on social media. Your words should not bully, harm, or insult. Cultivate a vocabulary that will allow you to express yourself exceptionally without the use of profanity. This unhindered ability will gain respect in any setting.

In this day and age of overt bullying and targeted verbal assassination of character, neither the perpetrator nor the recipient wins. Public ridicule about weight, skin color, overall appearance, and other particular attributes has caused an increase in the incidence of teen suicide. Don't be a source of detriment for others. Be their light by representing His light.

Things to Remember

_____

_____

_____

_____

_____

_____

_____

_____

_____

_____

_____

_____

_____

_____

_____

_____

_____

Things to Remember

Things to Remember

_____

_____

_____

_____

_____

_____

_____

_____

_____

_____

_____

_____

_____

_____

_____

_____

_____

_____

_____

Things to Remember

_____

_____

_____

_____

_____

_____

_____

_____

_____

_____

_____

_____

_____

_____

_____

_____

_____

_____

Things to Remember

II. The Heart

---

1 Corinthians 13:4-8, NKJV

"Love suffers long and is kind; love does not envy; love does not parade itself, is not puffed up; does not behave rudely, does not seek its own, is not provoked, thinks no evil; does not rejoice in iniquity, but rejoices in the truth; bears all things, believes all things, hopes all things, and endures all things. Love never fails."

The heart of your temple literally sustains life. It can move approximately five to seven liters of blood per minute and seventy-six liters (two thousand gallons) per day. It is a muscle. To work optimally, it needs exercise. As a teen, this is the ideal time to really figure out how to incorporate a healthy lifestyle into your everyday activities.

When I grew up, it was rare for me see adults in my family, in my neighborhood, and in my church attempt to exercise. As children, we were always sent outside to play, something that is less common today. Unsupervised bike riding, playing hide and seek, riding big wheels, jumping rope, and playing tag were ridiculously common. Few of us had a formal involvement in sports prior to high school. We were exercising almost daily unintentionally. That was plenty.

Nowadays, in the social media and digital game age, you are less likely to go outside unless you participate in a competitive sport. You'll need to plan to incorporate movement as medicine for your heart to keep it working at its best. It is God's center of His temple. The heart is a priority in self-maintenance.

The heart is also a symbolic center for love. Love comes in a variety of forms. You can love God, your parents, siblings, and grandparents. You can also love pets and other things that you are passionate about. Statistically, your first crush is not likely to be your life partner, although high school sweethearts may argue otherwise. At some point, you may be lucky enough to find one person to love for the rest of your life in marriage. God loves the church, and He is very clear about what love looks like.

Love is kind. Love is not jealous. It is not rude. It doesn't harm or wish harm on anyone. Love grows where there is truth not lies. Love endures; it's in it to win it. It is teamwork. Love sees the big picture while attempting to survive the small forest fires in the relationship. The one adjective God does not use to describe love is "perfect." Even amidst the imperfections of relationships, love is not violent. If you find yourself in an unhealthy partnership, cover it in prayer, tell a confidant, and make moves to keep yourself safe. Ask for help.

> You are loved.
> You are adored.
> You have value.
> God is love.

"I hope the next person who loves you takes you somewhere nice, and I don't mean lavish restaurants or on a costly vacation. I mean I hope they take you to parts of yourself you haven't yet seen. I hope they never drag you ankle first into your insecurities. I hope they don't shame you with the weapon of your past. I hope they trace your skin and show you where the light comes through. I hope they make you feel beautiful in the morning. I hope they walk barefoot inside of you. I hope they light candles just to see clearly. I hope they make you cider and you can tell them of the places you've been, the rubble, the dirt, the barb wired people it took for you to get here. I hope they carry you softly. I hope they take you somewhere nice."

—Sabah Khodir

Things to Remember

_____

_____

_____

_____

_____

_____

_____

_____

_____

_____

_____

_____

_____

_____

_____

_____

_____

_____

Things to Remember

_____

_____

_____

_____

_____

_____

_____

_____

_____

_____

_____

_____

_____

_____

_____

_____

_____

_____

Things to Remember

Things to Remember

_____

_____

_____

_____

_____

_____

_____

_____

_____

_____

_____

_____

_____

_____

_____

_____

_____

_____

_____

_____

_____

Things to Remember

III. The Lungs

Job 33:4, NIV

"The Spirit of God has made me; the **breath** of the Almighty gives me life."

In medical school, we are taught the ABCs for management of emergencies:

A - Airway
B - Breathing
C - Circulation

These are ranked in order of priority. Basically, what that means is that without a patent airway and breath, patients won't survive. Breath gives life. It is evident when a baby is born and takes his first breath. Life at its fullest begins.

If this component of the temple gives life, why would we want to damage it with inhalation of detrimental chemicals such as tobacco, cocaine, marijuana, and other unclean drugs? No illegal drug has been found safe over the years. Today's street drugs have been known to be filled with chemicals not designed for human ingestion or inhalation.

Eighty-five percent of lung cancers are due to long-term tobacco smoking. The remainder are caused by genetic factors, second-hand smoke, or exposure to asbestos and radon gas. Smoking cigarettes used to be considered "sexy." Today, with so much data revealing how addictive and dangerous nicotine has proven to be, more people are quitting the habit or at least trying. Vaping has been pinned as a safe alternative to traditional cigarette smoking because the nicotine used in these electronic cigarettes is vaporized rather than burned for inhalation. These e-cigarettes still contain the addictive substance nicotine, chemicals such as formaldehyde, in addition to flavor chemicals with unknown long-term sequelae. That's because there are no long-term studies comparing vaping versus traditional cigarettes and their effect on cancer prevalence or other potential health issues. If you have any lung disease, asthma included, you should not be using any inhaled substance unless it is a medication for your condition. Remember ABC- Airway, Breathing, Circulation. Nicotine affects all of those in a negative way.

According to the Center for Disease Control, "Cigarette smoking is the leading cause of preventable disease and death in the United States, accounting for more than 480,000 deaths every year, or about one in five deaths." In 2016, more than fifteen of every one hundred U.S. adults aged eighteen years or older (fifteen and a half percent) smoked cigarettes. This means an estimated 37.8 million adults in the United States currently smoke cigarettes. More than 16 million Americans live with smoking-related diseases. Smoking prevalence is decreasing over the years but the numbers of people still smoking is significant.

A smoking habit with more potent drugs usually begins with marijuana usage. This drug is not regulated for recreational use, so the chemicals are not consistent. This is the same for other street drugs as well. My recommendation to you is to avoid all illegal drugs, whether inhaled, being taken in pill form, or injected. You also should steer clear of any over-the-counter chemicals or drugs that are experimentally used in inappropriate ways. Again, use your common sense.

Use your breath for good. Because breath gives life, it also can be channeled for deep-breathing techniques to manage stress. Deep breathing for meditation and relaxation can provide healing effects. It's a free coping mechanism to use for alleviating anxiety about exams, driving, and dealing with tension. Learning how to meditate has huge health benefits. You will sleep better when it's done at bedtime. Meditation in the morning sets the tone for the day. You can't go wrong with that.

Be thankful for the breath the Almighty gives you daily, especially if you're breathing on your own. Somewhere someone is requiring a machine to assist them with breathing. Don't waste your blessing.

Things to Remember

_____

_____

_____

_____

_____

_____

_____

_____

_____

_____

_____

_____

_____

_____

_____

_____

_____

_____

Things to Remember

_____

_____

_____

_____

_____

_____

_____

_____

_____

_____

_____

_____

_____

_____

_____

_____

_____

_____

Things to Remember

Things to Remember

Things to Remember

_____

_____

_____

_____

_____

_____

_____

_____

_____

_____

_____

_____

_____

_____

_____

_____

_____

_____

_____

_____

IV. The Breasts

Genesis 49:25, NIV

"Because of your father's God, who helps you, because of the Almighty, who blesses you with blessings of the skies above, blessings of the deep springs below, blessings of the breast and womb."

I can't begin to tell you how many patients I have seen who have had concerns about the uneven size of their breasts. No one's breasts are exactly the same size, unless they've had some type of cosmetic surgery. Having one breast slightly larger than the other is the norm. No intervention is needed.

Invest in properly fitting bras. At your age, you don't have fifty-dollar breasts, so stick with more reasonable purchases. Realize that over time the bras will stretch out of shape, and your size may change based on fluctuations in your weight. Get sized by a professional. Sizing is free at some large department stores and lingerie stores. Make sure you own a strapless bra, a taupe bra to wear under white clothes, and a skin tone bra, or black bra.

If you are not adopted, please do your best to learn your family's female health history. Inform your provider of anyone with breast, uterine, ovarian, cervical, or other abdominal cancers. There are genetics screening tests that look for genetic markers that may indicate an increase in your risk of these cancers. Preventive measures can be taken to decrease your risk if you carry a predisposing gene. Surgical treatment options can also be reviewed.

Breast cancer is the most common cancer in women. Examine your breasts monthly, looking for unusual lumps that don't go away. Breast cancer is usually detected by a mammogram or palpable breast lump. A mammogram is a radiology procedure that takes pictures of your breasts to screen for non-cancerous and cancerous abnormalities. You do not need to have your first mammogram until age forty unless you have a significant family history.

Things to Remember

_____

_____

_____

_____

_____

_____

_____

_____

_____

_____

_____

_____

_____

_____

_____

_____

_____

Things to Remember

Things to Remember

Things to Remember

_____

_____

_____

_____

_____

_____

_____

_____

_____

_____

_____

_____

_____

_____

_____

_____

_____

_____

_____

Things to Remember

V. The Stomach

---

1 Corinthians 10:23, KJV

"All things are lawful for me, but all things are not expedient: all things are lawful for me, but all things edify not."

One perk during the teenage years is the uncanny ability for many to eat virtually whatever they want and not have to worry about weight gain due to a much faster metabolism than adults. Some, however, suffer from the opposite phenomenon, resulting in childhood and young adult obesity. Food choices for many are just that – choices. However, not everyone has the luxury of choosing to eat healthy foods on a regular basis. Access to proper food options require a number of factors: a nearby grocery store or market with fresh food and fruit as opposed to fast food restaurants or prepackaged meals, money to purchase the items, in addition to the knowledge and will power to choose healthier options that may not be a quick-fix. After all, it is much easier to go through the drive-thru for a burger and some fries, as opposed to making a home-cooked meal. How many teens do you know who can actually cook? Exactly – not many.

It has been shown that your waist measurement is a direct correlation to your overall health. Make exercise a lifestyle. Be active. Get outside with friends. Pull yourself away from your phone or TV and get moving. Being involved in a sport is supportive of healthy living, but simply walking or just riding a bike is great. Find something you enjoy, so it becomes part of a routine that can be modified through adulthood. You may not be fortunate enough to continue playing a competitive sport well into adulthood, but you should still be incorporating some form of exercise as part of a healthy lifestyle. Thirty minutes of cardio three to four times per week is recommended.

Too much of anything good can be bad. I love pound cake, my mother's version of sweet potato pie, bread pudding, Girl Scout Trefoil cookies and of course, Haribo gummi bears in the gold bag. I love sour gummi bears, worms, alphabet letters, cherries, basically anything Haribo. I have a difficult time not eating an entire sleeve of Girl Scout Trefoil cookies at one time. Believe me I get it when it comes to food kryptonite. It's okay to indulge at times. Overindulgence is never good when it comes to food. There must be balance. Try to tip the side of the scale that consists of healthy food choices including meat, fish, and vegetables heavier than the other side that consists of sugary and other high calorie foods like pizza, chips, candy, ice cream, and other goodies. Moderation is key.

SIXTH SENSE

If something is suspicious, beware and keep your guard up. This can apply to relationships and career decisions. Learn to trust your gut, which is also known as your sixth sense. Those butterflies or that sick feeling you get in the pit of your stomach may signal issues or trouble; pay attention to that. Instincts are God-given signals that need no explanation by facts. Many times, instinct stands alone as an urgency for decision-making. It can take years to learn how to fully tune in to those subtle feelings that provide direction for navigating life's problems. Honing that ability can save you from danger, relationship drama, projecting you towards decisions that will allow you to be the best version of yourself. Listen to it. Master it. The sixth sense should not be ignored.

Things to Remember

_____

_____

_____

_____

_____

_____

_____

_____

_____

_____

_____

_____

_____

_____

_____

_____

_____

Things to Remember

Things to Remember

Things to Remember

_____

_____

_____

_____

_____

_____

_____

_____

_____

_____

_____

_____

_____

_____

_____

_____

_____

_____

_____

Things to Remember

_____

_____

_____

_____

_____

_____

_____

_____

_____

_____

_____

_____

_____

_____

_____

_____

_____

VI. The Lady Parts

MENSTRUAL CYCLES

I'm confident someone in your family or church has encouraged you to protect your lady parts. That's great! What would be even better is understanding what those parts are supposed to do, how to appreciate what they were created for, and how to keep everything healthy. You need to know what is considered normal, so you can recognize abnormal conditions when they occur.

The most obvious body change for females is menstruation. It is called many things – most commonly your "period." The average age for a girl to get her first period is age twelve.

It can occur as early as age ten or as late as age sixteen to be considered within normal range. It's not uncommon for the frequency of periods to be irregular when they first start. If you have less than four periods per year, or if you're older than sixteen years old and still haven't gotten your period, please seek an evaluation by a medical provider.

A normal period (actual bleeding) should last no more than seven days. A normal menstrual cycle lasts anywhere from twenty-one to thirty-five days. A cycle consists of counting from the *first day of bleeding in one cycle* to the *first day of bleeding in the next cycle.* Many females inaccurately count from the last day of bleeding of one cycle to the first day of bleeding of the next. In other words, day one of your cycle is the first day of bleeding. This is key when trying to determine days for ovulation and figuring out when to expect the next cycle.

An average menstrual cycle is twenty-eight days long; therefore, periods cannot come on the same *date* of the month every time because months have different numbers of days. It is best to mark the first day of bleeding on a calendar each month. Average the number of days each full cycle lasts to predict a date for the next cycle. Always carry sanitary products with you in case your period gets thrown off schedule.

Did you know that you can get pregnant as soon as you start getting your menstrual cycles? In theory, you can even get pregnant before your very first period. During each cycle, the lining of the uterus, your womb, grows in preparation for a potential fertilized egg or embryo to implant. The egg is released from one of your ovaries monthly in a process called ovulation. Ovulation occurs day twelve to fourteen for those with twenty-eight-day cycles, or twelve to fourteen days before the next cycle. This egg is grasped by the end of a fallopian tube and moved down towards the cavity of the uterus. If the egg gets fertilized by a sperm and progresses to an embryo, that embryo implants into the plush lining of the uterus to begin growing into a baby. The uterine lining continues to grow; hence, there are no periods when pregnancy occurs. The majority of the time, however, the egg is not fertilized by a sperm so the lining sloughs off in the form of your period every month.

FEMALE REPRODUCTIVE SYSTEM

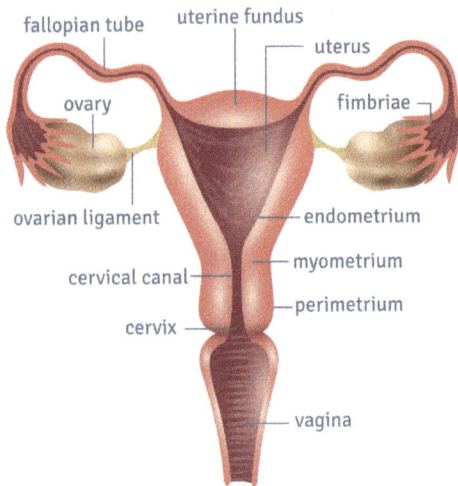

During your period, be sure to change sanitary products on a regular basis to reduce odor and infection. Consider products with all-natural fibers and minimal fragrance to minimize irritation. Try various sizes of pads and liners to determine which ones fit your body best. If you feel you're ready to try tampons, start with the smallest ones first. Larger tampons expand significantly and can be more difficult to remove once soaked. It's okay to wear a tampon and pad together. Just remember to change them in a timely fashion.

Pads come in a variety of sizes and shapes, some with wings and others without. There are even brands geared toward teens and athletes to better accommodate their smaller body types. You can experiment with regular and overnight brands of sanitary napkins. The overnight ones tend to be longer to cover more of your underwear to help prevent accidents. Try wearing dark panties during your period to minimize the appearance of blood stains. Wash them in cold water as soon as they get stained, so the blood will come out easier.

PERIOD PROBLEMS

Sometimes pain during your period, dysmenorrhea, may require medication for relief, or you may even need to miss days of school or work. If this is recurrent, please make an appointment with your pediatrician or an obstetrician gynecologist (OBGYN) to discuss remedies. An OBGYN specializes in caring for only females. Dysmenorrhea can be treated with heating pads, pain medicines, or hormonal medications. Talk with your doctor to figure out which remedy would be best for your condition.

Heavy, frequent, and unpredictable periods can also be managed with hormonal medications. The most common form of hormonal medications used to treat menstrual irregularities is actually contraception. There is an array of options for treatment including pills, patch, injectables, and implants. Final decisions on treatments may be based on your ability to be compliant with a regimen. You should really be open with your doctor about any concerns about being consistent with your treatment.

Please be honest when discussing your family history with your provider. Some genetic predispositions prevent you from using certain hormones. We don't want to cause harm. Every medication is not suitable for everyone. Please know that in most cases you do have options. You don't have to suffer.

COMMON INFECTIONS

Let's face it, sometimes the lady parts just don't smell fresh. Usually, it's because an infection is created by something you may have done differently. What's most important is knowing exactly where your infection is located. You have three openings in your genital area – one for water, one for blood and babies, and one for waste. Many females think they only have two. If you do have only two, that's a problem. I have had only one patient with that anatomical anomaly, and it required a complex surgical repair. You need to be aware of your orifices to become more knowledgeable about what is normal and abnormal in your body.

Your clitoris is the little pink sensitive area at the very top of your genitalia. Underneath that is a very tiny opening called the urethra. That opening leads to your bladder, which holds urine in the lower part of your belly. Urine comes through your urethra. It may be tricky to find. The easiest way for you to find it is by sitting on a commode and holding a mirror in front of your genitals. Spread your labia (the flimsy skin on both sides) and begin to urinate. You'll notice that the urethra is in close proximity to the vagina below it. This is why urinary tract infections (UTIs) are more frequent in females who are sexually active. Bacteria from the vagina can easily get into the urethra causing the infection. It's a good habit to urinate after intercourse to flush out any bacteria that may have entered the urethra during the process.

The urinary tract includes the urethra, bladder, ureters, and the kidneys. The ureters connect the bladder to each kidney. Symptoms of a lower urinary tract infection (UTI) include foul-smelling urine, frequent urination, pain or burning with urination, and urinating small amounts with incomplete emptying of the bladder. If the infection is severe, you may actually see blood in the urine. Untreated lower urinary tract infections can ascend to the bladder and even progress up through the ureters to the kidneys where urine is made. Your kidneys are located on both sides of your back right underneath the bottom of your ribs. Back pain and fever are the common symptoms of kidney infections, also known as pyelonephritis or shortened and called "pyelo."

UTIs are treated with antibiotics. A clean catch urine sample should be submitted for a urine culture. A urine culture determines the actual type of bacteria causing the infection. It also shows which antibiotics the bacteria are sensitive to and precisely how sensitive the bacteria would be to various medications. This allows the doctor to determine the best antibiotic to use for treatment. You should take the entire number of antibiotic pills prescribed for complete resolution and to prevent reinfection with the same bacteria.

Common vaginal infections occur when bad bacteria or fungus in the vagina out-grow the good bacteria in the vagina, which are there for protection. Yeast infections tend to produce a white, cottage cheese-like discharge in your underwear. The yeast can cause itching, and it smells like sour milk. The infection may be caused by taking anti-biotics for other infections. It can result from using fragrant soaps, vaginal products such as spermicide on condoms, or medical con-ditions that change the vaginal ph. Wearing wet bathing suits for long periods of time and tight clothing that doesn't allow the vagina to breathe can increase the occurrence of yeast infections. They may be treated with over-the-counter medications. If those are not suc-cessful, seek a prescribed medication from a medical provider.

Bacterial vaginosis (BV) is another com-mon vaginal infection that is not sexually transmitted. This infection has a classic fishy odor. There really are no over-the-counter treatments for BV. If you suspect you have this infection, you must be prescribed a vaginal or oral treatment by a medical provider.

INTIMACY

God has created the institution of marriage as the safe place for intimacy. As an OBGYN, I also realize that life happens, and many do not wait until marriage occurs to experience that sacred experience. As our Father, He knows that there are emotional connections, physical effects, and long-term sequelae that occur when engaging in sexual intercourse. He wants to keep you safe.

The brains of boys mature at age twenty-five, and girls' brains mature around age twenty-one. This, by no means, promotes dating someone four years older than you. Instead this information is given to explain who you're dealing with in the teen years. At age eighteen, you're only half way through the brain maturation process that started with puberty. The prefrontal cortex area in your brain is not completely developed. This part of your brain inhibits impulses and helps you organize and plan strategies to reach your goals. In addition, the brain's reward system becomes highly active at puberty and tapers off in the early twenties. This makes young people interested in risky situations to see if they can gain anything positive from the experiences. The story of the teen years and young adulthood involve hindered impulses and suboptimal decision-making techniques. Add sex to the mix and that creates a recipe of the "blind leading the blind" in some cases. God created you. He knows your body's limitations at this age ergo His fatherly advice on the topic of sex (NPR, Brain Candy).

If you are considering becoming intimate with someone or if you already have, here are a few pearls of knowledge. First of all, sex is not bad. God had to design something that would allow the world to continue to be populated. It had to be something enjoyable in order for procreation to continue. Sexual intercourse involves the male penis entering the vagina followed by ejaculation of a liquid called semen from the penis. The liquid contains sperm, which travel up through the cervix into the uterus, then through the fallopian tubes to fertilize an egg released from the ovaries. During intercourse, some couples attempt to practice withdrawal prior to ejaculation as a form of birth control. This, however, is not always effective because the small amount of fluid that leaks prior to actual ejaculation contains sperm as well. Additional forms of contraception (birth control) should be considered if pregnancy prevention is the goal.

Intimacy should occur between two *consenting* individuals, preferably adults. If you are an unmarried teenager being approached for intimacy by someone older than eighteen-years-old, you should know the laws in your state. Statutory rape occurs when a person over the age of consent has sexual intercourse with a person under the age of consent. The age of consent varies by state. In some states the age is sixteen, and in others, the age is eighteen. Breaking the law can result in unnecessary charges when violations are discovered.

Regardless of your age, if you find yourself in a situation where you do not want to proceed with having sex, your "no" always means "no." Any act of sex after your declaration of "no" is considered rape. Alcohol and other drugs can impair proper decision-making. Be intentional in keeping yourself unharmed by not allowing yourself to enter those situations in the presence of mind-altering drugs. Report any wrongdoing immediately. Sex can be used as a tool of power – even as an adult. Make your intentions and desires known. You have a voice in the matter.

If you have found someone you feel will be a long-term partner, form a strong friendship first. Do not succumb to pressure to have sex to keep him. That decision should be discussed thoroughly. This partner should be someone who is not only attracted to you physically but also to your mind, your ambitions, and your goals in life. He, too, should have life goals. He should not be abusive. Teen domestic violence is a real phenomenon. He really should be someone who makes you better.

Keep in mind that you are to protect the one place in this world that can grow and produce a human being. Nothing else has the ability to create a human life in its fullest viable form. Hopefully, if you are seriously contemplating intercourse, you have a trusted adult in your life who can assist with this life-changing decision. This sacred area of your temple should be guarded from misuse, infections, and even cancers. Be proactive about keeping it safe from harm.

INFECTIONS AND CONTRACEPTION

With sex comes more complex decisions about relationships and prevention of pregnancy. As a teenager, having a baby is not an optimal situation. Abstinence is ideal. Condoms help prevent pregnancy but have the highest failure rate of all birth control methods. The rhythm method or ovulation tracking may work for those with very regular cycles. The following contraception options have the lowest failure rates for preventing unwanted pregnancy:

1) Daily -taking an oral contraceptive pill

2) Weekly - using a patch

3) Monthly - using a ring inserted inside of the vagina

4) Every three months – an injection

5) Every three years – an implant on the inside of your upper arm

6) Every three to five years – an intra-uterine device (IUD) placed vaginally inside the uterus

7) Every ten years – an intrauterine device placed vaginally inside uterus, sometimes can make your periods a bit heavier

Oral contraceptive pills (OCPs) require timely compliance to be effective. It's best to simply set a daily alarm on your phone as a reminder. The time for taking your pill should be a time you can be consistent with even on the weekends. If you miss a pill or take it late, it loses its contraception efficacy, and you are likely to have some type of breakthrough bleeding during the month.

Birth control that is weekly or monthly allows for less maintenance. OCPs (daily use), the patch (weekly use), and the vaginal ring (monthly use) allow flexibility with the frequency of periods. Their usage can be manipulated such that periods can be spaced to every three months or longer without harm.

The arm implant and intrauterine devices require the least amount of maintenance and are the most effective forms of reversible birth control. The IUDs are placed by a medical provider in an office. It is not a major surgical procedure by any means. After placement, there is a string that hangs through the cervix not outside of the vagina like a tampon. IUDs are perfect for females in mutually monogamous relationships who are not potentially exposing themselves to any sexually transmitted infections (STIs). Rarely, STIs such as chlamydia can become attached to the IUD string, travel up into the uterus and out through the fallopian tubes, causing a syndrome called pelvic inflammatory disease (PID). This can potentially impair fertility, your ability to get pregnant in the future. Your provider may want to screen you for chlamydia and gonorrhea prior to IUD placement.

STIs

The most common symptom of a sexually transmitted infection is no symptom at all.

Condoms can also help prevent transmission of sexually transmitted infections, but unfortunately, they cannot prevent them all. Be sure you are current with your vaccinations, particularly for the human papilloma virus (HPV) that can cause genital warts, cervical, oral, rectal, and penile cancers. If you are sexually active, you should get screened for infections at least yearly. Condoms only cover the penis. Contact with other parts of the male genitalia can expose you to other infections such as genital warts and herpes simplex virus.

Gonorrhea and chlamydia are screened by placing a cotton swab in the vagina in the opening of the cervix and underneath the cervix. It can also be screened with a urine sample. If you have decided to risk other sexual practices, be sure to inform your doctor so those areas may be screened as well. Herpes is screened by sampling an active sore. Diseases such as HIV, hepatitis and syphilis must actually be detected with bloodwork.

Most times males discover they have an infection because their partner was diligent about her healthcare and got tested. If they are fortunate enough to actually have symptoms, they usually seek medical treatment. However, as previously mentioned, the most common STIs tend to be asymptomatic. Also realize that most infections are spread because the carrier had no idea he or she was infected. When you get tested at the doctor's office, you're actually testing both you and your partner. Untreated infections such as chlamydia can decrease fertility later in life. Infections such as herpes and HIV are life-long.

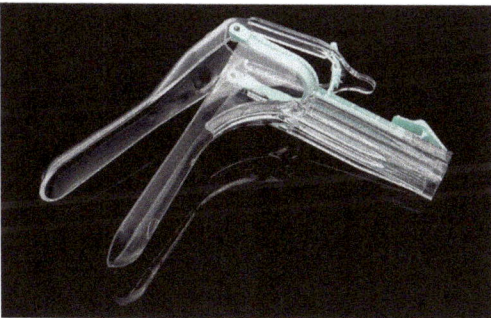

GYNECOLOGICAL EXAM

Your first gynecological (gyn) exam can be daunting. It will consist of a physical examining of your lungs, breasts, abdomen, internal and external genitalia, and your rectum. The provider will have you complete a health questionnaire to get a detailed personal medical history and family history. This examination may occur close to home with your pediatrician or an OBGYN. Perhaps it will occur while you're away at college. Never lie to your doctor when responding to questions. Your answers could save your life. For example, if you have a family history of blood clots, you may not be a candidate for medications with the hormone estrogen. Disclose all pertinent information even if you feel embarrassed. Female health concerns, history of a sexually transmitted infection, sexual practices, sexual abuse, and domestic abuse are all topics that can be shared with your doctor in private.

A thorough bilateral breast exam will be performed. Some patients say it tickles, but it is completely painless. Your doctor will also show you how to check your own breasts. A pelvic exam will then be completed to screen your cervix, uterus, and ovaries.

If you are at least twenty-one-years-old, a pap smear will be performed. A pap smear is a screening test for cervical cancer and precancerous changes in the cervix. The procedure is slightly uncomfortable. A plastic device called a speculum is gently inserted inside of the vagina. A plastic brush is used to obtain cells from the cervix. There is no cutting or snipping. If the results are normal, the American College of OBGYN recommends that this test be performed every three years. The pap smear can also test for gonorrhea and chlamydia in some cases. If you are younger than twenty-one-years-old and sexually active, your doctor will still place the speculum to visualize your cervix, but only STI screening will be performed rather than a pap smear. It is best not to decline this testing if you are sexually active. Remember, you are getting screened for both you and your partner. Be diligent with your healthcare.

Contraception options will be offered as well as additional screening by bloodwork for other STIs such as HIV, hepatitis, and syphilis. You need to know your own health status before getting involved intimately with someone. Detailed testing should be performed particularly with new partners, suspicion of cheating by your partner, and at least yearly if you are not in a long-term, monogamous relationship. Take care of your temple.

Things to Remember

Things to Remember

Things to Remember

Things to Remember

Things to Remember

Conclusion

Jeremiah 29:11, NIV

"For I know the plans I have for you," declares the Lord, "Plans to prosper you and not to harm you, plans to give you hope and a future."

As you mature into a bold, God-loving, young woman, you will come across questions about your body that simply spark curiosity in addition to questions that may require answers from a medical professional. God created an amazingly complex temple for each of us to use while here on earth. As females, our temples are even more spectacular because they are the only creations, specifically made by Him, to bring forth human life. I encourage you to educate yourself as much as possible about this masterful machine. You are the operator of this exquisite vessel. Protect it. Operate it with much care.

There's a saying that you can't soar with the eagles if you're running with the turkeys. Your village should encourage and motivate you, help you dream bigger. Find your village and love them hard. Surround yourself with a few "ride or die" friends. This will not be a large number because these people will become a part of you. First of all, they should love Him. They may call Him by a different name; however, they appreciate that there is a power greater than themselves that governs their hearts and moral compasses. These friends will hold you accountable for your actions, listen to your ideas, tell you honestly if they are absurd or dangerous, get you through your first heartbreak, and laugh and cry with you. They should want to protect you and cause no harm. You should be inspired by them. They should spark joy for you and you should do the same for them.

My prayer for you is that you fill your temple with positive energy and thoughts of Him, that your life's vision be made crystal clear, and that you have discernment of people and situations around you to protect your mind, heart, body, and soul. Allow your head to overflow with positive thoughts, imagery, and words that move you forward on the path God has orchestrated just for you. You may not always stay precisely on that path, but you will no doubt be able to find your way back on task if you keep your eyes on Him. I pray God builds your village circle to only include those who are for you and about Him. And lastly, I pray that you remain safe during your quest of educating yourself on all topics, especially those about your own body. May He provide answers of light for you in safe spaces, so that you may go forward and be a light for the world.

Amen.

Sources

About the Author

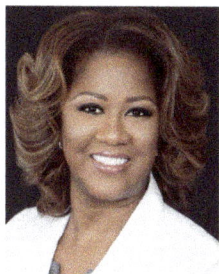

Dr. Suleika Just-Buddy Michel is a board-certified obstetrician gynecologist with twenty years of experience whose ministry is educating females about their bodies. As the first African American partner in her OBGYN practice, she is a well-respected advocate of minimally invasive surgery and is a trained DaVinci robotic surgeon. Inspired by her mother, who was a registered nurse, Dr. Michel always knew she wanted to enter the medical field. She is the first physician in her family.

After realizing her children's Christian elementary and middle schools had no formal health education for students, she decided to create a faith-based health curriculum specifically for preteen and teen girls in fifth through twelfth grade. She now holds seminars for local schools and churches throughout Maryland discussing female health from a biblical perspective. Her goal is to provide a safe space for girls to be educated with age-appropriate information about their bodies.

To learn more, visit
DrSuleikaMichel.com

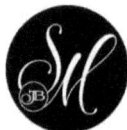

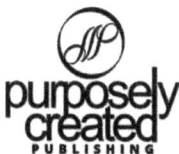

CREATING DISTINCTIVE BOOKS
WITH INTENTIONAL RESULTS

We're a collaborative group of creative masterminds
with a mission to produce high-quality books to position
you for monumental success in the marketplace.

Our professional team of writers, editors, designers,
and marketing strategists work closely together to ensure
that every detail of your book is a clear representation
of the message in your writing.

Want to know more?
Write to us at info@publishyourgift.com
or call (888) 949-6228

Discover great books, exclusive offers, and more at
www.PublishYourGift.com

Connect with us on social media

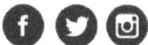

@publishyourgift

www.ingramcontent.com/pod-product-compliance
Lightning Source LLC
Chambersburg PA
CBHW042248040426
42336CB00043B/3364